HONEY

THE HONEY WONDER

The Many Wonders Of Natural Honey For Beauty, Healing, Natural Cures, Cooking And Lots More

LOLA CROSS

ISBN-13:978-1508966074
ISBN-10:1508966079

Disclaimer

The information in this book is solely for informational purposes, not as a medical instruction to replace the advice of your physician or as a replacement for any treatment prescribed by your physician. The author and publisher do not take responsibility for any possible consequences from any treatment, procedure, exercise, dietary modification, action or application of medication which results from reading or following the information contained in this book.

If you are ill or suspect that you have a medical problem, we strongly encourage you to consult your medical, health, or other competent professional before adopting any of the suggestions in this book or drawing inferences from it.

DEDICATION

To God, for creating bees

TABLE OF CONTENT

INTRODUCTION

Honey—The Wonder Food

Honey is a pure and natural sweetener that has been consumed by man for centuries. Every year, the honey bees produce about 1 million tonnes of honey worldwide. Of this number, 285 million pounds are consumed by Americans alone.

Honey is a wonder food. It is one of the healthiest, most delicious and sustainable sweeteners in the world. It never seems to go bad, develop mold or contaminate even when it is not refrigerated after being opened. Archeologists reportedly found 2000-year old honey jars in Egyptian tombs and they were still fresh and tasted delicious!

Since bacteria love sugar, isn't it surprising that they cannot grow in honey? The reason is that honey is a natural antibiotic. It has a unique chemical composition of relatively high acidic level and low water content that creates a low pH environment, making it extremely unfavorable for bacteria to grow.

Think honey if you wish to enhance your health and that of your household. Its natural healing characteristic will help to control diabetics, cholesterol levels and blood sugar. This way, your body will heal faster than any supplements options in the market.

Honey has proven it can strengthen the immune system so it should be part of your daily diet (the darker, the better). It certainly makes sense to have a little raw honey every day because it will not only make you feel more energetic, but also help you to stay healthy.

However, do not give raw honey to children under the age of one as it contains the spores of botulinus. Infants who are of this age may not have the required stomach acid to stop these spores from developing. This may lead to botulism, a life-threatening disease.

Two Common Honey Varieties

While there are several honey varieties available, for the purpose of this book, we would consider Manuka and Raw honey, which are acclaimed for their extraordinary health benefits.

Manuka Honey

Made in New Zealand, Manuka honey is obtained from the nectar of Manuka flowers. Unlike other honeys, it contains an additional, naturally occurring active ingredient which is stable and sustains its potency even when it is exposed to light, heat or dilution. It has been clinically tested for wounds, herpes blister and skin ulcers treatments, It stimulates tissue healing.

Manuka honey can be used in treating many types of ulcers, post-surgical wounds, abscesses and fistulas. It is also used in treating non-healing wounds in cancer patients, as well as those induced by radiation therapy.

Raw Honey

Raw honey is the most original honey that the honeybees produce. It is honey that has not been heated or filtered. It contains small quantities of the same resins that are found in propolis. When extracted, the honey is warm and flows with ease. Consuming local raw honey provides you with immunization against allergies.

The Many Wonders Of Honey

It Is Nutritious.

Honey contains several vitamins like B6, riboflavin, niacin, thiamin, pantothenic acid and some amino acids and minerals such as copper, calcium, iron, magnesium, phosphorus, potassium, manganese, sodium and zinc.

It Is A Very Healthy Food Choice.

Honey's sugar absorb gently into the blood stream, resulting in better digestion.

It Energizes.

Honey is a natural carbohydrate source that provides the body with strength and energy. It helps to boost the performance and endurance of athletes.

Since it contains natural fruit sugars, glucose and fructose, it is able to prevent fatigue during exercises.

Additionally, honey contains no cholesterol thus including small quantities of it in the daily diet helps to keep the cholesterol levels in check.

It Builds Immunity Against Sicknesses And Diseases.

Honey contains antioxidants that help in eliminating free radicals and biologically harmful chemical agents that cause diseases like cancer.

It strengthens white blood cells and promotes blood formation. Honey also helps to supply the nutrient needed for the growth of new tissue.

It Beautifies You.

Honey has hygroscopic properties so it can be used as part of natural beauty recipes for skin care, hair care, facial scrubs, moisturizers and skin care.

It keeps the skin fresh and hydrated. With its natural anti-microbial and antioxidant properties, it rejuvenates and refreshes the skin, making it soft and supple.

It Acts As A Natural Remedy For Many Health Problems

Honey is the only natural sweetener that has healing effects. A wide range of health problems and ailments can be effectively treated with honey as you will soon discover in this book.

Medicinal Properties of Honey

Antibacterial

Antioxidant

Anti-allergic

Antiviral

Anti-inflammatory

Autoimmune protection

Eye health

Wound healing

Promotes calcium and selenium absorption

Prebiotic effect promoting healthy gut

Honey: Myth & Fact
Fact

• Honey is sweeter than table sugar

• Honey's quality or nutritional value is not affected by crystallization.

• Honey is a healthier option compared to artificial sweeteners.

• Honey contains zero cholesterol

• Honey helps your body to burn fat even while you are asleep

Myth

• Honey should never be scooped with a metal spoon —
although honey is acidic; the action of scooping honey
takes just a few seconds so corrosion cannot even occur.

• Honey is best mixed with hot water —adding hot water
to honey reduces its aroma and flavor and may also
destroy a few healthy enzymes that are contained in it.

• Honey never spoils, even when stored in an open jar —
if honey is left uncovered for an extended period of time,
it will absorb moisture from the air and this will lead to
fermentation.

• Honey can be bought in powder forms — natural honey
is only available in liquid forms and cream but not in
powder form. Cactus honey powder should not be
mistaken for natural honey as it is not produced by bees
but from the juice of the agave cactus plant.

• Honey contains a little fat — this is untrue. Honey is
100% fat free

Cooking with Honey — Practical Tips

• Honey is nearly twice as sweet as sugar so use less of it when cooking.

However, some honey varieties like Tupelo are sweeter than others.

• When cooking, replace 1 cup sugar for ½ cup honey. Honey also attracts water so reduce liquid quantity by 1/4 cup for every cup of honey added to the recipe.

• When baking, compared to sugar recipes, beat vigorously and for longer. Honey batter also becomes crisper and browns faster too. Simply lower the oven temperature by 25degree F.

• To neutralize the acidity of the honey, add 1/2 teaspoon of baking soda for each cup of honey. This will also help the food rise.

• When making use of honey in jellies, jams, or candies, raise the cooking temperature a little so that the extra liquid will evaporate.

• Honey has a way of enhancing, balancing, or imparting its flavor to other foods so consider its floral variety when cooking with it. The large number of mouthwatering recipes with honey that are available today is due to the many honey varieties and the versatile ways they are cooked.

Have These Cooking Qualities Of Honey At Your Fingertips:

• Extends shelf-life — a natural preservative for sauces and pickles.

• Enhances flavor — an excellent natural sweetener for cold beverages and hot teas.

• Provides feel and texture — a great addition in cake making and pastries.

• Adds color — contributes an agreeable golden hue to jellies, dressings, sauces and frozen desserts.

• Retains moisture — a vital ingredient that provides the moisture in quality cakes and prolong the moisture retention.

• Binding viscosity — a wonderful ingredient that helps the shaping of desserts like cakes, pastries and puddings.

Measuring Honey Accurately

Baking or cooking with a large quantity of honey can be messy and confusing. Learn how to get the precise measurement neatly and correctly.

1. Brush or smear the inside walls of a measuring cup with baking/cooking oil thinly and evenly all around it.

2. Pour the required amount of honey into the measuring cup.

3. The thin and even layer of oil makes it impossible for the honey to stick onto the cup.

4. You can now pour out the honey from the cup and none will be stuck to the measuring cup. Also, you do not need to scrap out the remaining honey from the measuring cup so as to obtain the accurate amount of honey as required in the recipe.

HONEY TREATMENTS FOR BEAUTIFUL SKIN

Honey treats blemishes effectively and helps the skin to retain its moisture. As a natural antiseptic, Honey is just right. It is the ideal ingredient for masks and cleansers. It will moisturize and condition your face, leaving no trace of oil.

Honey & Egg White Mask

1 tbsp honey

1 egg white

1-2 drops tea tree oil

Instructions:

1. Mix ingredients together. Apply on face and let it stay for 10-15 minutes.

2. Rinse face with warm water.

3. Refrigerate left over mask for up to 1 week

4. Use mask 2-3 times a week

Face Mask For Acne

Cinnamon exfoliates and will stimulate your pores. Nutmeg will even your skin tone and work as an anti-inflammatory as well. Lemon juice removes dead skin cells and aids fade scars.

3 tbsp honey

1 tsp cinnamon

1 tsp nutmeg

Lemon juice (optional)

<u>Instructions:</u>

1. Combine all ingredients in a small bowl until dark brown and slightly thick.

2. Refrigerate mixture to further thicken and make application easier.

3. Apply mixture to face, leave for 30 minutes, rinse and dry gently. Moisturize if needed.

4. Refrigerate the rest.

Pore Refining Toner
1 tbsp honey

2 tbsp witch hazel

1 tsp lemon juice

Instructions:

1. Combine ingredients. Let it sit for 3-4 days before using. This way, the honey loses its stickiness.

2. Refrigerate toner.

Rejuvenating Facial Mask
1 tbsp honey

1/4 cup dried apricots

1 tbsp dried milk

¼ cup water

Instructions:

1. Blend ingredients with electric blender.

2. Leave on face for 15 minutes. Rinse thoroughly.

Anti-Aging Skin Care Recipe
This recipe fights hydration. The honey will draw out skin impurities and moisturize naturally. This makes it the ideal ingredient for a homemade anti-aging skin care recipe.

1. Cleanse your skin. Apply 1tbsp honey all over the face.

2. Leave it for 10 minutes. Rinse off with warm water.

3. Add a tablespoon of brown sugar for extra exfoliating power

Honey Complexion Brightener

Equal part honey

Equal part Lemon juice

Instructions:

1. Mix together and apply to face and neck.

2. Leave it for 5-10 minutes then rinse.

Natural Skin Polisher

1tbsp sugar

11/2 cup honey

Instructions:

Mix together and use 2-3 times a week

HONEY TREATMENTS FOR HEALTHY HAIR

Honey contains potassium as well as vitamins A, B and C. These nutrients keep the hair healthy, moisturized, and shiny. Thus, it is the perfect treatment for conditioning hair. Use these honey hair treatments regularly as a preventative measure, for dry and brittle hair, to repair damaged hair as well as for color-treated hair.

Garlic – Honey Scalp Treatment

Garlic increases blood circulation to the scalp, helps to reduce hair loss and prevents dandruff. Honey protects the hair and makes it smooth and silky.

1/2 cup honey

Head of garlic

Shampoo Hair conditioner

Instructions:

1. Cut up cloves with cheese grater or mash in a garlic press.

2. Combine the honey and garlic in a bowl.

3. Using only your finger tips, rub this mixture into your scalp and hair. Do this for 5 minutes.

4. Rinse hair with warm water, wash with shampoo and then apply the conditioner.

5. Rinse with cold water to have a shiny hair.

Anti-Hair Loss

When it comes to treating hair loss, honey is a dependable natural ingredient. It will make your hair follicles really stronger.

1. Massage 1 tsp honey into your scalp. Let it stay for 1 hour then rinse off.

2. It can also be mixed with hair shampoo or conditioner.

Hair Strengthener

1 tbsp honey

½ cup olive oil

Instructions:

Mix and apply to the hair. Let it stay for 30-45 minutes then rinse off.

For Brittle Hair (caused by dry weather conditions)

1 tbsp honey

1 egg yolk

1 tsp olive oil

Instructions:

1. Mix together to make a rich hair conditioner

2. Use 1-2 times weekly

Hair Mask
Restore color, body and shine to your hair

1. Apply1/4 to 1/2 cup pure honey onto hair and wrap hair in plastic.

2. Leave honey-saturated hair on for 25 minutes. Rinse off

Hair Removal Wax
To remove hair effectively, honey wax must be kept at the right temperature. If it is too cold, it will create a difficult and sticky mess on your skin. If it is too hot, it could cause skin irritation or burns.

1 cup honey

1 cup white sugar

Juice of ½lemon

Instructions:

1. Combine sugar and honey in a small electric pot. Add lemon juice.

2. Set electric pot to low temperature, cover and cook for 2 hours. The honey should be thin and the mixture should be easy to stir using a flat wooden stick.

3. Leaving the electric cooking pot still on, remove lid for about 10 minutes for wax to cool for a while before you begin waxing.

4. Using a flat wooden stick, scoop up some wax and carefully touch it with your finger tip to ensure it is cool enough to use.

5. In a 4-inch long by 2-inch wide strip, spread the wax onto the desired skin area.

6. Next, press a strip of cotton fabric that is larger than the wax strip onto the warm honey wax. Smooth down the cotton strip by using your hands to rub it firmly 3-4 times.

7. Hold the skin around the strip firmly with one hand. Using the other hand to grasp the edge of the cotton strip, pull it off quickly in the opposite direction of the hair growth.

8. (Your hand should be very close to the skin when pulling off the strip so you wouldn't cause yourself unnecessary pain).

9. Keep applying and removing the wax the unwanted hair has been completely eliminated then gently wash the skin with warm water to remove any leftover wax.

10. Do not use lotions or soap as they may irritate your newly-waxed skin.

Honey Hair Rinse
For healthy and shiny hair

1tsp honey

4 cups very warm water

Instructions:

1. Combine ingredients and transfer to a plastic squeeze bottle.

2. Shampoo the hair and then apply this treatment to the scalp and hair.

3. Let it stay on for 2-3 minutes then rinse with warm water.

4. For best results, let the hair air dry. Use daily.

Honey Banana Deep Conditioner

This powerful solution coats the hair cuticles, resulting in locks that are healthy and manageable.

1 ripe banana, mashed

1tbsp pure honey

Instructions

1. Combine ingredients until a smooth consistency is achieved.

2. Next, dampen the hair with warm water. Take the mixture and massage it onto the hair and into the scalp.

3. Cover the hair with a clean towel, shower cap or plastic wrap and leave for 20 minutes before rinsing.

4. Shampoo and condition for the hair to air dry. Use it at least twice a week.

Honey Olive Deep Conditioner
3tbsp honey

1tbsp olive oil

Instructions:

1. Mix together until smooth. Shampoo hair and apply the mixture to it.

2. Let it stay for 15 minutes. Use warm water to rinse.

3. Apply once in a week. For very long hair, double the ingredients.

HONEY FOR MEDICINAL PURPOSES
Keep your body hydrated once you have a cold so that the congestion caused by the virus will be loosened with no difficulty.

COUGH SYRUPS
Honey-Lemon Cough Syrup

This very common homemade cough honey recipe is easy to make and highly effective for soothing sore throats and mild coughs.

16 ounces raw honey

1 lemon

Instructions:

1. Place the honey in a pan then cook on low heat but do not let it boil.

2. Bring a separate pan of boiling water to a boil, place lemon in it and leave to boil until the outer skin becomes soft. Leave to cool. Slice the softened lemon into 4 pieces.

3. Place the sliced lemon into honey and simmer on low heat for 1 hour. Pass mixture through a strainer to remove seeds and lemon. Let the mixture cool.

4. Once cool, place in a container, cover and put in the refrigerator for up to 2 months.

5. Take 4 times daily or as needed. Adults-1Tablespoon; children 50 pounds and above-1 teaspoon; and children under 50 pounds - ½ tablespoon.

Anise-Honey Cough Syrup

Anise helps to treat coughs, asthma and bronchitis.

2 cups honey

1 tsp anise seed, crushed

Instructions:

1. Bring 1½ cups water to a boil, place the crushed anise seed inside, cover and set aside for 30 minutes.

2. Pass liquid through a strainer, simmer until 1 cup remains then add honey and mix thoroughly.

3. Place in a sealed container and refrigerate. (Can last up to 2 months)

Horehound-Honey Cough Syrup

Horehound contains a phlegm-loosening expectorant. It is extremely effective in the treatment of coughs and colds.

Honey

1 ounce horehound leaves, dried

Instruction

1. Bring 16 oz water to a boil then place the horehound leaves in it. Let it sit 10 minutes.

2. Strain to remove the leaves. Next, add one part of the mixture to two parts honey, shaking thoroughly.

3. Place in an airtight jar and refrigerate for two months. Take 4 times daily or as needed.

Honey Gargle For Sore Throats
For quick relief

3 tbsp raw honey

1/2 tsp cinnamon powder

1 cup hot water

Instructions

1. Mix ingredients together.

2. Gargle with this mixture 4-5 times daily to soothe your sore throat.

Or:

2 tbsp honey

4 tbsp squeezed lemon juice

Pinch of salt

Instructions

1. Mix ingredients together.

2. Gargle with this mixture 4-5 times daily to soothe your sore throat.

Honey Cough Drops
Natural, sweet and very effective!

1 cup raw honey

1 tsp cinnamon powder – optional

Instructions:

1. Boil honey to 300 degrees F. Pour mixture into small candy molds or drop 1/2 tsp amounts onto parchment paper.

2. Leave to cool completely before removing from parchment paper or molds. Enjoy!

Natural Flu Shot
Taste sour but works like hell!

3 tbsp raw honey

Juice of 6 lemons

3 cups Pineapple Juice

1 clove of garlic

1/4 tsp cayenne powder

Instructions:

1. Blend all the ingredients and store in a jar.

2. Take 1 cup four times daily until all symptoms disappear

Garlic& Honey Cold Treatment
Garlic and honey are natural antibacterial ingredients that fight cold-causing germs and boost the immune system.

½ cup raw honey

4 garlic cloves, peeled & sliced into 8 pieces

Juice of 1 lemon

Instructions:

1. Place garlic pieces in a saucepan, add 4 cups distilled water to it and bring to a boil on medium-high heat. Once mixture emits a garlic scent, remove from heat.

2. Add honey to garlic water, stir and add lemon juice to the mixture.

Arthritis Honey Remedy

Lemon helps to lessen the inflammation that causes arthritis.

1tsp honey

1 cup warm water

1-2 tsp lemon

Instructions:

Mix well and drink 5-6 times daily

Bad Breath Remedy (halitosis)

Get rid of the bacteria that cause bad breath with this effective remedy and enjoy fresh breath from day to day.

1tsp honey

$\frac{1}{4}$ tsp cinnamon powder, ground

11/2 cup hot water

Instructions:

Mix the first two ingredients in the hot water and gargle 2 times daily.

Athlete's Foot Remedy

This common foot problem is caused by fungus growth and can be treated by a common remedy- Honey.

1. Apply a generous amount of honey on the affected area and rub thoroughly.

2. Wear an old pair of socks to cover feet before going to bed.

3. The following morning, wash feet off and dry.

4. Continue this treatment until the problem disappears.

Rosacea

Treat the blemishes and redness that accompanies Rosacea with honey.

Raw honey

Little amount of distilled water

Instructions:

Mix together, apply to the face and leave for 3 hours or leave overnight.

Generally, redness and blemishes of Rosacea are difficult to treat, so be patient.

Burns

This treatment helps to prevent infections, redness and blisters. This is highly effective when the burn is immediately treated.

1. Apply a thin layer of honey on the burn and let it stay for 30 minutes. Wash off.

2. Apply to the affected area twice daily until the burn has healed.

3. Keep the area clean at all times to speed up the healing process.

Gum Disease

Clear up gum problems. Prevent them as well.

Instructions:

1. Brush your teeth. Massage honey on the gums for 5 minutes.

2. Do these 2 times a day. Alternatively, dilute honey with water and use as mouthwash

3. Additionally, you could add it to your toothpaste.

Eczema

No matter how stubborn or difficult your eczema, honey's several healing properties can handle it well.

Equal part honey

Equal part cinnamon

Instructions:

Mix and apply to affected area.

To prevent recurring eczema:

1 tsp honey

Juice of half lime or lemon

Instructions:

Add ingredients to 1cup water. Stir well and drink.

Eye Infection

Eye infection is caused by bacteria and thus can be treated with honey.

Equal parts honey

Equal parts distilled water

Instructions:

1. Mix and apply to eye with a cotton ball.

2. Leave on the eye for 30 minutes or apply as eye drops to the eye two times daily until the infection disappears.

Sinus Infection

Manuka honey destroys the germs that affect the sinus, throat and nose.

1 tsp Manuka honey

1/4 tsp baking soda

1/4 tsp sea salt, non-iodized

1 cup distilled water

Instructions:

1. Bring distilled water to a boil, add Manuka honey and stir. Next, add the baking soda and salt to it.

2. Let the mixture cool then pour it into a sterile container. Cover and refrigerate

3. using a sterile eye-dropper, apply the Manuka honey mixture by drawing it into the dropper, tilting your head back, and dispensing 8- 10 drops into the nostril.

4. Repeat as needed throughout the day.

5. For preventative purpose, take 1 teaspoon of Manuka oil orally every morning.

Note: Do not use Manuka honey if you suffer from bee sting allergies, tuberculosis, heart conditions or bee sting.

If you are diabetic, see your doctor about the required dosage that is safe for you.

Indigestion

Honey promotes the growth of probiotics like Acidophillus and Bifidus which are essential for good digestion. It also helps to reduce stomach acid and quickly too.

1. Honey and lemon. Mix and drink.

2. To calm stomach, add honey to herbal tea.

Upset Stomach

With this remedy, your stomach troubles will be gone in no time.

1 tbsp honey

1 cup warm water

¼ tsp ground cinnamon

Instructions:

Add honey to warm water, mix well then add cinnamon to it.

Drink on an empty stomach

Ulcers (stomach and mouth)

Stomach ulcers are caused by Helicobacter pylori bacteria. Honey's antibacterial properties can help in treating this problem.

Instructions

1. Take 1 tbsp raw honey thrice daily with or without water.

2. It works for mouth ulcers as well.

Warts
1. Apply honey to wart then apply gauze on it.

2. Apply fresh honey daily until warts and scars disappear.

3. This can take up to 2 weeks.

Yeast Infection
1. Apply honey over affected area.

2. Let it stay for at 10 -15 minutes then rinse off.

3. Do this twice daily, in the morning and at night before bedtime.

HIDDEN WONDERS OF HONEY YOU NEVER THOUGHT OF

Honey Nail Strengthener
Get smooth, polished and stronger nails with this remedy

1 tbsp honey

¼ cup milk

2 egg yolks

Instructions:

1. In a small bowl, beat egg yolks and add milk and honey.

2. Place your nails inside this mixture for 10 to15 minutes.

3. Rinse your hands under cold running water and pat dry.

Get Rid Of Stress
The antioxidants in honey help to reduce stress levels.

1 tbsp honey

3 tbsp of warm water

Instructions

Mix ingredients, sip slowly and feel the stress disappear.

Sleeplessness/Insomnia
Having trouble sleeping? This remedy should help. It is extremely soothing and has a calming effect.

1 tsp honey

1 cup warm milk

Instructions

Combine and drink.

Honey For Insomnia: How It Works

Insomnia is dangerous for both children and adults because it comes with severe consequences such as mood swings, lack of concentration, obesity and severe health-related issues.

Nightly honey consumption leads to a little increase in blood sugar level and this leads to a controlled rise of insulin. When this happens, tryptophan, a sleep-promoting amino acid enters the brain. It gets converted to serotonin, a relaxing hormone. Now, once it gets dark, the serotonin converts to melatonin, which is widely used to cure sleeping disorders such as insomnia.

Another way that honey eliminates insomnia is by reducing stress hormones production at night. The body stores its energy source (glycogen) in the lever. Nevertheless, the liver may run out of glycogen at night.

When this happens, the brain triggers stress hormones like cortisol and adrenaline and the body will then be able to convert the protein muscle into glucose. The good thing is that honey is the best food for glycogen storage due to its ratio of fructose to glucose which is 1:1.

Asthma Relief

Asthma is caused by a variety of factors such as environmental conditions and allergies. However, honey offers tremendous relief.

1tsp honey

11/2tsp cinnamon

Instructions:

1. Mix well and consume. Alternatively, add mixture to 1 cup warm water.

2. Remedy is best taken before going to bed at night.

Memory Zest Blend

A mentally refreshing beverage for clarity and precision

Honey

1 part ginkgo

1 part rosemary leaves

1 part peppermint leaves and gotu kola

1 part ginger root

1 part red clover tops

Instructions:

1. Bring an entire tea pot or cup of water to a boil. Add the herbs.

2. Let the tea steep for 10-15 minutes, strain and add honey and drink.

Honey Lavender Lip Balm

1/2 tsp raw honey

1 tbsp shea butter

2 tbsp coconut oil

2 tbsp beeswax

1 tbsp sweet almond oil

5 drops Frankincense essential oil

15 drops Lavender essential oil

<u>Equipment:</u>

1 large rubber band

12 lip balm tubes

<u>Instructions:</u>

1. Take the lids out from the lip balm tubes and then secure them upright with the rubber band.

2. In a double boiler, gently melt the honey, coconut oil, beeswax and shea butter.

3. Take out from heat. Add the essential oils and sweet almond oil then stir.

4. Pour the melted oil immediately into the upright tubes.

5. Let the lip balm to set then close the containers.

Honey for Hangover
Honey calms the effects of the alcohol on the body and eliminates any cravings.

1. Upon waking, take 3-5teaspoons of honey. Depending on the severity of the hangover, keep on with this dose every 20 minutes.

2. At breakfast, take 4 more teaspoons.

Detoxification

Cleanse your system with:

21/2 tsp honey

1 lemon wedge

Instructions:

1. Add honey to I cup of boiling water. Stir well to dissolve.

2. Add the lemon wedge and drink.

Improve Your Immune System

Boost your immune system to be stronger against bacterial and viral attacks with:

2 tbsp honey

1 tsp cinnamon

Instructions:

Mix well and take.

Honey For Weight Loss

Take this drink when on a diet and when you crave something sweet.

1 tsp honey

1/2 tsp cinnamon powder

1 cup water

Instructions:

1. In a small saucepan, mix all three ingredients together.

2. Bring the mixture to a boil. Allow it to cool then refrigerate.

3. Take half of cup of this mixture 1 hour before breakfast. Take another half cup 1 hour before bedtime.

Tip: How Honey Works For Weight Loss

Honey is a natural energy-giving food. It works as a fat burner so it can be used as part of a recipe for weight loss. Sugar is highly processed so the nutrients benefits are minute, if at all in existence.

1 tsp sugar = 16 calories

1 tsp honey= 21 calories

Therefore, honey has a healthier glycemic index when compared to sugar. Thus when honey is consumed, it absorbs gradually into the body, providing you with a source of stabilized energy. You will not experience that energy crash or a sugar "high" afterwards.

Honey is also sweeter in taste compared to sugar. For this reason, less honey is needed. It is also more flavorful so add only a little to your food and drinks. Just a little bit of honey will satisfy you. This will keep you from cheating on your diet.

For individuals who are on a diet, exercising self control becomes easier to achieve. Simply take a little bit of honey and your 'sweet tooth' will be effortlessly satisfied. Honey helps with the low energy levels experienced by most people on a diet. With honey consumption, your energy level is stabilized all through the day.

Honey For Lower Cholesterol
Bad cholesterol (LDL) levels can now be lowered with honey as honey contains lots of antioxidants which stops plague from accumulating on blood vessel walls.

1tsp honey

1 cup warm water

Instructions:

Mix well and drink daily

How Honey Lowers Cholesterol In The Body
Cholesterol is essential to several human functions. For instance, it helps to produce many hormones that are used in several cell membranes. In spite of its significance, high

cholesterol is risky to the heart and likely to cause heart attack.

The wonders of honey in lowering cholesterol in the body

Honey contains nutrients that fight the cholesterol in the body. Calcium, sodium, potassium and vitamin B complex are a few of these nutrients. Honey also contains antioxidants that help in increasing the level of blood within the body especially when it is taken daily.

It can also help to clean the blood vessels consequently lowering the chances of high blood pressure in body. This is definitely better than any health enhancement supplements available.

Honey For Diabetes Solution

Honey does not raise blood sugar levels in the same way table sugar does. Therefore, diabetics are usually advised to eat foods that contain plenty of vitamins C, E, B1, B12, B6 as well as Biotin.

All these nutrients can be found in any good quality honey.

Honey For Exercise

Exercise is important to keep fit and for weight loss. When you eat honey, you get the needed energy. Research has shown that athletes who eat some honey after their performance recover faster. Reducing heart attack incidences becomes easier as well.

So get into the habit of taking a little honey when going to the gym or going for a walk. You will be able to endure vigorous exercises

Instructions:

1. 1 tsp of raw honey added to your water bottle is all that you need.

2. You will feel real good after the workout.

FORMS OF HONEY

Freezing Honey

Freezing honey is the best way to store it. Overtime, honey ages and loses its color and flavor. Honey should never be refrigerated as it will change flavor and granulate and you may eventually have to throw it away.

Instructions

1. Divide the honey into small amounts as it is pointless to freeze the entire bottle then thawing it all when needed.

2. Freeze honey in a sealed glass container. (Plastic container may affect the flavor of the honey).

3. Place a label with the freezing date of the honey neatly pasted on it. This will help you to know the container of honey to use first.

4. Don't remove the honey from the freezer until you are ready to use it. Give the honey plenty of time to thaw.

Preventing Crystallization Of Honey

Crystallization is the process of solidifying honey. Honey that is kept in the freezer will not solidify as a result of its low moisture content. Glucose content in honey is less soluble than fructose so it will crystallize when it is separated from the water.

To dissolve the crystals, the honey can be placed in the microwave but it is better to prevent crystallization completely.

Freezing honey prevents crystallization, although it may have to be thawed before it can be poured easily.

Things You'll Need

Honey

Plastic wrap

Ice cube tray

Instructions

1. Pour the honey into an ice cube tray. (A larger container should be used if you are using large amounts of honey at the same time).

2. Use the plastic wrap to wrap the ice cube tray or container and then place in the freezer. The honey will become very thick but will not freeze. (The plastic wrap

stops other freezer odors from entering into the honey. Also, if the tray tips, the freezer will remain clean).

3. Remove the number of cubes that is needed, leave them to thaw on your counter or place them straight into your recipe. Each cube holds about 1 tablespoon.

4. An entire honey container can also be frozen; defrost for 30-40 minutes before using.

Hardening Honey

Honey eventually hardens or crystallizes naturally due to small particles of sugar, wax, crumbs or pollen that enable the honey crystals to form.

Crystallization doesn't mean that the honey has gone bad. As a matter of fact, honey stored in a cool environment when opened remains fit for human consumption for at least 10 years. Unopened honey is indefinitely edible.

Some people enjoy crystallized or hardened honey because the water content evaporates and this intensifies the sweetness. However, if you cannot wait for the honey to crystallize naturally, cook it to a toffee-like consistency then make lozenges.

Things You'll Need

1/2 cup honey

2 cups sugar

1 tbsp vinegar

1/4 cup water

Double boiler

Instructions

1. Pour water in the bottom of a double boiler then bring to a boil. Lower heat

2. Add water, honey, vinegar and sugar in the second pan and place it into the boiling water. (The sugar allows the honey to crystallize when the solution cools).

3. Bring second pan to a boil. Reduce to a simmer. Constantly stir so it doesn't stick.

4. Once the solution gets to about 300 degrees F, carry out a hard-crack test. Fill a glass cup with cool water. Add a spoonful of the honey into the water to cool. The honey should immediately snap when you remove it after cooling,

5. If it bends or rolls into a ball before breaking, keep heating and do the test again after 1- 2 minutes.

6. Take out the pan of honey from the double boiler. Divide the thickened honey before it cools.